Hormone Replacement Therapy: The Truth About HRT

The Ultimate Beginner's Guide to Hormone Replacement For Women and Men

Table of Contents

Introduction

Menopause is an issue facing everyone, both men and women. The aging process is inevitable, and menopausal symptoms will soon affect each individual. The symptoms can be mild, almost like a minor daily discomfort. In some, the symptoms may turn so severe that a person needs to be confined to bed for a few days. However, life in your later years does not have to be spent suffering. To address menopausal discomforts, HRT was developed.

This short and concise book provides introductory information on HRT treatments and how they may help people. The content here isn't meant to be a form of medical advice, as this book is meant for informational purposes only. In this book we are aiming to look at this topic in an unbiased light. We are not promoting the use of HRT, per se, but we want to make sure that if someone is interested in this controversial topic, he or she can reach more informed conclusions.

We will discuss the history of HRT, the science behind it, and how it can affect one's body. Most practically, we will look at the pros and cons of this medical treatment and how it compares to other options out there.

We hope that you are able to learn a thing or two from reading this!

Chapter 1:

What is Hormone Replacement Therapy?

As a person ages, several things change in his or her body. One in particular is the significant change in the levels and proportions of a person's hormones. The imbalance starts off with a decrease in the production of the hormones estrogen and progesterone. This change sets off an imbalance in the entire body, which increases a person's risk for several ailments, such as stroke, blood clots, diabetes, and cardiovascular problems.

Hormones in the body interact in a well-coordinated manner. Changes in the levels of one hormone will cause other hormones to adjust. However, during menopause, the decline in progesterone and estrogen levels is rapid, giving very little time for the rest of the hormones to adapt. Also, the rapid decline places the rest of the body's organs in a mad scramble in order to compensate, resulting in forms of discomfort such as hot flashes, mood swings, and irritability. This state also places the rest of the body at a higher risk for numerous health problems.

HRT, or hormone replacement therapy, seeks to resolve this hormonal imbalance. It aims to bring back the normal levels of estrogen and progesterone. By keeping these hormones within the normal range, the rest of the body gets to achieve homeostasis and things go on as usual.

Types of Hormone Replacement Therapy

Estrogen and progesterone are derived from non-human sources and then administered to an individual. Estrogen used in HRT comes from plant estrogens, such as from a certain species of yam, or extracted from a pregnant horse's urine. Progesterone in HRT is synthetic (produced in laboratories), which is called progestogen. The human body easily absorbs this synthetic progesterone replacement.

Estrogen-Only

One of the three basic types of HRT is the administration of estrogen only. This is usually the most recommended type of HRT for women who have undergone a hysterectomy - the surgical removal of the uterus (womb). This type is usually not used because of its high risk for the development of uterine cancer (cancer of the womb) or endometrial cancer. Nonetheless, for those who have already had their uterus (womb) removed, estrogen-only HRT is fine because there is no longer any threat of developing endometrial cancer.

Cyclical HRT (aka Sequential HRT)

In this type, estrogen and progesterone are administered. This is most recommended for women who are in the menopausal stage but are still having their menstrual periods. There are to two kinds of cyclical HRT: monthly or quarterly.

In the monthly HRT, estrogen is taken every day. Progesterone is taken only for 12 to 14 days, towards the end of the menstrual cycle. This is more appropriate for women who are still having regular menstrual periods.

The quarterly HRT is similar to the cyclical HRT, but only the schedule of progesterone is modified. Estrogen is still taken on a daily basis. Progesterone is taken for a period of 12 to 14 days. However, instead of monthly, progesterone is taken every 13 weeks. This type of HRT is recommended most for women who have irregular periods. In the quarterly HRT, the woman should have her period every three months.

The cyclical HRT is very useful in maintaining regular periods throughout the menopausal stage. This will help in finding out when the period naturally stops and when the last stage of menopause is to be expected. It is important to note that a small number of women who undergo cyclical HRT report experiencing continued regular periods even after menopause.

Continuous Combined HRT

This type of HRT is more advisable for postmenopausal women - women who have not had any periods for at least the last twelve months. Estrogen and progesterone are taken on a daily basis, without any breaks.

Contraception

Estrogen taken in HRT is not the same as the estrogen taken for contraception. Hence, a woman can still get pregnant while on HRT. Some women can be fertile even up to two years after she has had her last menstrual period. This is especially so if she was just under 50 years old when she had her menopause. For women who had their menopause after 50 years of age, they can still be fertile for a year after their last period.

If not wanting to get pregnant at this time, then non-hormonal contraceptive methods are recommended. Taking contraceptive pills that contain estrogen and progesterone are not advised. These can interfere with the action of HRT and vice versa. The desired contraceptive effects and the HRT actions won't be achieved. To avoid pregnancy, use diaphragms, condoms, and other non-hormonal means of contraception.

There is one hormonal contraceptive method, though, that can work with HRT. This is the IUS, or the intrauterine system. This is also given to women who have heavy periods. The IUS can effectively help avoid pregnancy and can act as the progesterone portion of HRT. Estrogen would just have to be taken via patch, gel, or tablet.

Indications for HRT

So, who can take HRT? Women who are at the early stages of menopause are recommended to start HRT if they are interested. They can begin HRT as soon as the early signs of menopause are experienced. Age varies, with an average age of 50 years old and beyond as the start of the menopausal period for women, and some experience symptoms as early as in their 30s or as late as in their 60s.

A few women experience early menopausal symptoms, such as vaginal dryness and hot flashes, a few years before they do get into their menopausal period. This typically happens about 3 to 4 years before the actual menopausal stages. This period is called peri-menopause. Some women experience peri-menopause because the number of their eggs (ova) drops below a certain level, causing a decline in the levels of their progesterone and estrogen levels.

Generally, a woman can choose to undergo HRT without having to test if she is indeed in the menopausal period. This is only necessary if the woman is younger than 40 years old or if she has experienced unusual bleeding patterns during her periods. The test is only done to rule out any other conditions that may be contributing to menopausal symptoms, such as hyperthyroidism.

Contraindications to HRT

People who have the following are not suitable candidates for HRT because of potential serious complications:

History of cancer involving the reproductive organs, such as cancer of the breast, uterus, or ovaries

History of clotting problems (prone to or had incidence of blood clot formation)

History of stroke or any heart diseases

Untreated high blood pressure (needs to be controlled before undergoing HRT)

Presence of liver disease

Pregnant

HRT and Men

Hormone replacement is most popular among menopausal women. However, men too can benefit from HRT. The primary difference is that, in men, the main hormone is testosterone instead of estrogen.

Testosterone is a very important hormone in men. It maintains the proper functioning of the different reproductive organs. It also provides supportive and protective effects on different tissues, such as development and maintenance of muscle mass, levels of red blood cells, and proper bone density. By the time a man reaches the age of 30, his testosterone levels steadily decline. This places a man at a higher risk for serious conditions, such as a stroke and diabetes.

The Issue

HRT is believed to be helpful in improving a man's testosterone levels. However, there is an ongoing debate as to whether HRT is indeed helpful. There aren't a convincing number of studies on the effectiveness of HRT in men. The few studies available are relatively small and the results are inconclusive. HRT to improve testosterone levels in men due to the effects of aging are yet to be clinically proven.

HRT is recommended for men who suffer from hypogonadism resulting in low testosterone levels. In this condition, the testes are not functioning properly and are not able to produce enough of the male hormone. For men undergoing HRT for hypogonadism, options include:

Testosterone replacements administered via muscular injections every 2 to 3 weeks,.

Testosterone replacements administered daily via patches, with areas of application rotated between the arms, back, abdomen, and buttocks.

Testosterone replacements applied via gel preparations and topically applied over the abdomen, arms, or shoulders.

In the United States market, there are no approved testosterone pills available at the moment. Because of the potential liver toxicity from adding testosterone this way, most people would rather not take the risk. Additionally, there haven't been any that prove to be effective at significantly increasing the levels of testosterone in men.

Chapter 2:

History of HRT

In the 1940's, HRT became available for women who were suffering from menopausal symptoms. Widespread use began during the 1960's, when HRT created a revolution in menopause management. It became a common prescription for relief of symptoms during menopause, such as night sweats and hot flashes, as well as sleep disturbances, vaginal dryness and urinary frequency. It was even used as a means of preventing the development of osteoporosis, which commonly develops when estrogen levels fall.

In America, Premarin was the very first HRT brand that became available to menopausal women. This was composed of CEE, or conjugated equine estrogen, a natural but nonhuman estrogen derived from the urine of pregnant horses. In the 1950's, there was a growing concern over this mode of treatment. Not too many people were comfortable with the idea of using horse estrogen to increase a woman's estrogen levels. Also, statistics had shown that a significant number of women undergoing HRT developed uterine cancer. After a few years, the company that manufactured Premarin was prompted to make some modifications to their product. They then developed the drug Prempro, which was similar to Premarin but had the hormone progesterone added to it.

In the next few decades, HRT became a standard prescription for menopausal women. HRT was advertised as a means of keeping aging women younger and to help them retain their femininity. It was also claimed to keep women's skin looking young, their bones stronger, and their mental capabilities sharp. More and more doctors were prescribing it to relieve menopausal symptoms such as mood swings, weight gain, hot flashes, and insomnia. In fact, within the medical field, doctors who did not prescribe HRT were considered to not be practicing good medicine.

In the 1990's, a resurgence of concern over the effects and the effectiveness of HRT resurfaced. One of the common concerns raised was in regards to the dosage. Women experienced different sets and varying degrees of menopausal symptoms, but the dosages were all the same. Another question arose regarding the source of the estrogen - the pregnant horse. The question was mainly about the condition of the pregnant horse. Also at this time, women were becoming more and more interested in alternative methods.

Breakthrough Study

However, even with these concerns, there were still a lot of women who believed HRT worked and swore by its effectiveness. There were still a significant number who were willing to undergo the treatments. In 2002, a breakthrough study was made by the WHI (Women's Health Initiative). The study involved an extensive evaluation on the effects of Premarin and Prempro as part of HRT. Both of these hormonal replacements were not bioidentical (same in composition, structure, and function as a woman's naturally synthesized reproductive hormones).

In the United States, the WHI conducted a randomized clinical trial. In the United Kingdom, another large study was done by the MWS (Million Women Study), which made use of observational questionnaires. Both of these studies raised concerns and put forward two main issues:

Extended or prolonged use of HRT can increase the possibility of developing breast cancer.

HRT may raise the risk of developing a heart disease.

The study included more than 16,000 women in the postmenopausal stage. The results were:

Doubled risk of dying from breast cancer among Prempro users compared to women who took placebo

Doubled death rate due to breast cancer among women who took combination drug that contained estrogen and progesterone compared to the group that took placebo

An overall 25% increase in risk of invasive types of breast cancer among users of non-bioidentical HRT

CEE use was linked to the reduction in the risk of hip fractures

Reduction in the risk of hip fractures and development of colon cancer among users of combined estrogen and progesterone therapy compared to placebo

Needless to say, these findings were overwhelmingly convincing and created a huge change in the medical community. The results established that HRT did not in any way reduce a woman's risk for heart disease. Instead, HRT definitively raised the chances of developing stroke, breast cancer, and blood clots.

There are still a few debates as to whether these findings are conclusive. One issue raised was in regards to the effect of HRT on younger women who were experiencing peri-menopause. Newer research found that there was a significant difference in the way HRT affects a 50-year-old woman placed on the therapy and a woman who had HRT at least 10 years after she had menopause.

With these results, more research was conducted. The participants in the WHI study are now being reexamined to see if there is any subset of women who experience benefits from HRT and if there is any subset of women who should be avoiding HRT. Each reanalysis of this WHI breakthrough study is hotly debated, with no conclusive results yet. What remains clear is that there is a difference in the response to HRT between women in peri-menopause and those who were 10 years postmenopausal. The risks are definitely less in women who are in a postmenopausal stage.

The result of the WHI 2002 study also created widespread confusion. Women who heard about the result immediately stopped HRT and sought alternative treatments. However, as soon as they stopped HRT, their menopausal symptoms came back. Women were faced with a dilemma - continue with HRT to control menopausal symptoms but suffer the risks or stop HRT and suffer menopausal symptoms. Disappointment was all around as women were at a loss regarding what to do. To add to this, companies that manufactured the drugs used for HRT maintained that there were no good alternatives to HRT.

Today, more and more women are discovering that there are natural treatments that can help with their menopausal symptoms. These natural methods can also help them in transitioning off of HRT.

HRT in the UK

When the results were published, regulatory authorities in the UK issued urgent safety restrictions on HRT. Doctors were recommended to prescribe the lowest possible dose effective for symptom relief. Also, the recommendation included that HRT be used only as a second line of treatment and for osteoporosis prevention. It was also highly advised not to use HRT in postmenopausal women that were asymptomatic.

One argument in the UK against the WHI study was that the participants were North American women, not from the UK. These women were mostly in their mid-60s and mostly overweight. These were not representative of the average woman from the UK in her menopausal years. In the UK, women experience menopause between 45 to 55 years of age - a much younger group than the ones who participated in the study. With this age discrepancy, some groups maintain that the WHI study results are not conclusive and certainly not applicable to the average menopausal group in the UK.

Also, a closer look at the WHI results found that most of the women who had increased risk for breast cancer were the ones who were already on HRT before they participated in the study. This meant that they were on HRT for a much longer period of time.

Another issue raised against this major WHI study was that age was a factor, although the authors of the study claimed age did not play an important factor. Further evaluation of the WHI study revealed that women who started HRT within 10 years after their last menstrual period had no increased risk of heart disease.

Furthermore, on the issue of risk of heart disease and HRT, another large controlled study was conducted in Denmark during 2012. This most recent study demonstrated that HRT did not increase the risk of heart disease in all women. Healthy women who took combined HRT for a period of 10 years right after their menopause experienced a lowered risk of heart disease.

This study paved the way for the concept of a window period for optimum HRT benefits. This result and conclusion is even supported by the WHI study, where women who started HRT by the age of

60 had an increased risk of heart disease. Therefore, if HRT is started right after menopause, then heart disease can be prevented. If HRT is started at a much later time, then the potential for heart disease is increased.

Chapter 3:

The Science Behind HRT

As mentioned earlier, HRT was basically developed in order to provide relief for menopausal symptoms, as these symptoms can become so severe that women can no longer enjoy life or even function normally. The decline in estrogen and progesterone promote discomfort and some medical problems that drastically reduce the quality of life. One example is osteoporosis, which puts a woman at a higher risk for hip fractures and other symptoms brought about by the accelerated loss of bone density.

Menopause

Menopause is an occurrence that comes with the natural aging process that all women and men go through. The severity of these symptoms varies among individuals. Some people experience these symptoms more frequently and more severely than others. Also, a person may find the symptoms to vary in intensity depending on days, overall conditions, and some other factors, such as stress and sickness.

Hot flashes are the most common menopausal symptom, which also gives one of the greatest discomforts during this period. It is a sudden hot feeling over the upper body, and possibly the entire body. Some women feel the heat over the face and neck, often resulting in a reddened appearance with flushed and sweaty skin, and hot flashes typically last anywhere from 30 seconds to 10 minutes.

Vaginal symptoms include changes in the lubrication and appearance of the vagina. Vaginal dryness is a common symptom, which can lead to painful sex because the vagina isn't producing enough lubrication from low estrogen levels. Depending on how severe the decline in estrogen levels are, the vagina may atrophy (shrivel up).

Why HRT?

Certain symptoms of menopause are relieved when the levels of reproductive hormones in the body are brought back up to the normal range. HRT basically works by increasing the levels of reproductive hormones that the body is no longer producing on its own in normal amounts.

For instance, estrogen replacements relieved the increased warm feeling in the upper body, as well as hot flashes. It also helps to relieve genito-urinary symptoms, such as vaginal dryness, itching and burning, and urinary difficulty and frequency. Estrogen replacements also help in slowing down the loss of bone density, or osteoporosis. However, estrogen replacement does not directly address other symptoms such as depression or anxiety. Also, progestin, the synthetic progesterone hormone, is added to HRT to reduce the risk for uterine cancers.

Direction For Use

HRT is typically taken once per day through tablets. Experts recommend taking the tablet at the same time each day. Prempro, FemHrt and Activella are all available as tablets. These contain both estrogen and progestin.

Ortho-Prefest is available in a 30-tablet blister card. One pink tablet contains estrogen only and is taken once per day for three days. One white tablet (contains both progesterone and estrogen) is taken once a day for three days. Repeat this schedule until all of the tablets in the blister card have been consumed. Right after finishing the last tablet, start another blister card.

Premphase is available in dispensers that contain 28 tablets. One maroon tablet contains estrogen only and is taken once per day from day 1 to day 14. One light blue tablet contains both progestin and estrogen and is taken once per day from day 15 to day 28. Start a new dispenser on the next day after finishing the previous dispenser.

Chapter 4:

The Effects of HRT

While it is generally safe, there are a few concerns over the potential side effects of HRT. These are synthetic hormones after all, even though some are from natural sources.

The side effects of estrogen and progesterone

Most often, these side effects get better with time. It is often only due to the adjustments that occur as these hormonal replacements work their action. The improvements usually become evident within three months after the initiation of HRT.

If these side effects persist beyond three months, check with a doctor and reconsider continuing with HRT. Expected options in this case include any of the following:

Switching method of administration. For instance, switching from patch use to oral administration with pills

Changing the current type of HRT. For instance, changing to a different form of progesterone, estrogen or testosterone

Adjusting the current dosage of HRT

Estrogen Side Effects

Commonly associated side effects of taking estrogen for HRT include the following:

Bloating

Leg cramps

Fluid retention

Headaches

Nausea

Swelling or tenderness of the breasts

Indigestion

Making a few changes in your lifestyle is often enough to get rid of these side effects, such as:

Taking estrogen with food helps in reducing indigestion and nausea

Modifying your diet to be low in fat and high in carbohydrates helps to relieve breast tenderness

Stretching and regular exercise helps to relieve leg cramps

It is very important to observe these side effects. Report to your doctor immediately if these side effects intensify or resolve over the following weeks, as these may indicate the development of complications.

Progesterone Side Effects

Progesterone replacements are associated with the development of the following side effects:

Breast tenderness

Acne

Mood swings

Fluid retention

Backache

Headache

Depression

Side Effects In Men

In men, the side effects are the main reasons that a lot are hesitant to undergo HRT. Some are minor, but there are also more serious ones. Minor side effects include:

Acne

Fluid retention

Increased urination

The more serious potential side effects include:

Decrease in the size of the testicles

Enlargement of the breasts, referred to as gynecomastia or "man boobs"

Infertility

Decrease in sperm count

Increase in red blood cell count

Changes in the levels of cholesterol

Worsening case of sleep apnea, if the man is already suffering from it before HRT was initiated

Prostate growth has also been observed in men who underwent HRT. Because of this potential side effect, men who have been diagnosed with prostate cancer, or are at a high risk for developing it, are highly discouraged from undergoing HRT.

Chapter 5:

The Pros and Cons of HRT

The debate regarding the effectiveness of HRT and the benefit to risk ratio still continues to this very day. Benefits include the effective relief of symptoms such as hot flashes and night sweats, reduced risk for osteoporosis and improved vaginal and urinary discomforts (i.e. vaginal dryness and urinary frequency). In women below 60 years of age who are taking HRT, protective effects against certain problems, like stroke and heart disease, are also provided. However, the major issue clouding all of these benefits is the huge risks.

Risks

Taking HRT is known to increase a person's risk for conditions such as:

Stroke

Blood clots

Heart attacks

Breast cancer

This is why it is very important to observe the side effects closely. For instance, persistent and unrelieved leg cramps may be an indication of blood clot formation within the leg veins. The lower limbs are a common site for blood clot formation because of its dependent position.

Persistent headaches may be a warning sign for an impending stroke. Unrelieved indigestion may be a warning sign that a heart attack is about to happen. Breast tenderness that does not go away has a slight possibility of an increased risk of a developing breast cancer.

Other considerations

For women who are considering starting HRT, consult and tell a doctor if you:

Smoke

Have breast lumps

Have blood clots

Have hypertension

High lipid profile

Are diabetic

Also, if you are about to undergo surgery, inform the surgeon. Estrogen and progesterone would have to be temporarily discontinued 4 to 6 weeks prior to most surgeries.

Immediately seek medical attention if the following side effects are experienced:

Sudden and severe headache

Sudden loss of vision, either partial or complete

Sudden and severe vomiting episodes

Sudden shortness of breath

Difficulty in talking

Faintness or dizziness

Heaviness over the chest or crushing chest pain

Numbness or weakness on one limb (arm or leg)

Pain over the calves

These are indicative of an impending stroke, blood clots, or heart attack. Seek immediate medical care.

Health and Safety Concerns

These hormones, although in slightly different formulation, do cause these side effects even when used outside of HRT. For example, contraceptives that contain estrogen, progesterone or a combination of both will still carry these risks. However, in HRT, there are more concerns over the health and safety risks of the entire method.

Advocates of HRT maintain that, while the method is not entirely risk-free, the benefits far outweigh the risks. They claim that HRT still remains to be the single most effective treatment for menopausal symptoms. In men, advocates still maintain that HRT is still more effective in restoring normal testosterone levels compared to other similar methods. Also, in certain groups, HRT is known to provide protective effects for the cardiovascular system against diseases.

Chapter 6:

HRT Compared to Other Hormone Therapies

HRT is not the only solution to problems regarding the balance of reproductive hormones in both men and women. There are also a few alternatives, such as the administration of bioidentical hormones, tibolone, antidepressants, and clonidine.

Bioidentical hormones

In more recent years, the emergence of bioidentical hormones is being recognized as a better and safer solution compared to HRT. Bioidentical hormones are hormones naturally synthesized by the human endocrine system, particularly by the ovaries, and specifically progesterone, estrogen, and testosterone. These hormones naturally decline once the ovaries stop releasing eggs during menopause.

Pharmaceutical companies in the 1990's started the development of different methods of administering bioidentical hormones. The most popular method was via a patch. The first of which was Climara. The hormone delivery system was via a sticky transdermal patch applied over the skin. One interesting thing about Climara was that the hormone itself could not be patented, even though it is similar in structure to human estradiol. It was only patented for the glue and not for the estrogen hormone it contained.

Studies have shown that the use of bioidentical hormones actually promotes a protective effect against certain diseases, such as breast cancer and heart disease, which are conditions that have an increased risk of developing with HRT.

Tibolone

Tibolone is a synthetic hormone that can be used instead of HRT. Women who still have their womb intact may opt for this kind of therapy. Tibolone consists of a mixture of estrogen and progesterone. This formulation reduces the need to take the female reproductive hormones separately.

Compared to HRT, tibolone therapy is more convenient and requires replacement hormones to be taken less frequently. However, the same side effects may be experienced. Also, contraindications for tibolone are the same as those for HRT. For instance, women who have a history of cancer of the reproductive organs, such as breast cancer, are also not advised to undergo tibolone therapy.

Also, unlike HRT, tibolone therapy is not recommended for women who are experiencing peri-menopause. Women have to wait a full year after their last menstrual period before they can take tibolone. This, for a lot of women, would mean having to deal with discomfort for a long time before they can experience the relief provided by tibolone.

Antidepressants

Antidepressants are also prescribed for women who are experiencing the negative effects of declining estrogen and progesterone. However, these drugs are not given to relieve hot flashes. Some of the common antidepressants given for menopausal women are citalopram and venlafaxine HCl. Side effects can be expected with the use of these drugs, such as:

Dizziness

Nausea

Dry mouth

Sleeping difficulties

Anxiety

Decline in sex drive (libido) in some women

These side effects should improve over time. If not, consult the physician for a change of dose or change of drug, or to stop use of the medication.

When taking antidepressants, close monitoring is very important. Regular blood tests are needed in order to test the blood levels of the drugs to prevent overdosing. Blood pressure monitoring is also very important, as there is a risk for hypertensive crisis or orthostatic hypotension while on antidepressants. These are crucial for women who are currently taking antihypertensive medications or anti-clotting drugs. These are also very important in women who suffer from hypertensive conditions.

Clonidine

This is an antihypertensive medication that can also help relieve menopausal symptoms. It can help reduce night sweats and hot flashes. This drug, however, can cause side effects such as:

Drowsiness

Dry mouth

Fluid retention

Constipation

Depression

A trial period of 2 to 4 weeks is needed to test if it is effective for an individual, as not all women respond well to clonidine. If after the trial period the symptoms are not effectively relieved, then treatment is discontinued.

Chapter 7:

The Future of HRT

Today, HRT is using safer hormone preparations. Also, close monitoring and working with physicians is very important in order to assess its effectiveness and prevent any serious complications from occurring. People undergoing HRT must be completely assessed by their physicians on a yearly and as needed basis.

Also, more people are coming back to HRT because there hasn't yet been anything that can provide the relief that HRT provides. More recent studies also found that HRT is safe for long-term use, such as for prevention of osteoporosis, as long as it is taken using the lowest effective dose.

Furthermore, risks are significantly lowered if HRT is started early, around the time when a woman first enters menopause. Starting within this period is crucial to reduce the associated risks with HRT use. Women over the age of 60 are not highly advised to undergo HRT but can still get the treatment as long as they receive the right monitoring and proper dosages. In case you were wondering, this does not mean that women who started early with HRT need to discontinue treatments when they reach 60.

The introduction of bioidentical hormones has made HRT even more effective and recommended. These still carry the risks and side effects of hormone replacements but on a much smaller scale.

Women can now enjoy their youthful femininity without having to worry about suffering serious complications later on in life. They also no longer have to suffer through menopause, and they can continue to live productive and satisfying lives as they please.

However, for men, there has yet to be more studies confirming if HRT is safe or if it is really effective in improving low testosterone levels due to aging. This benefit has not yet been fully explored and clinically tested to assure safety.

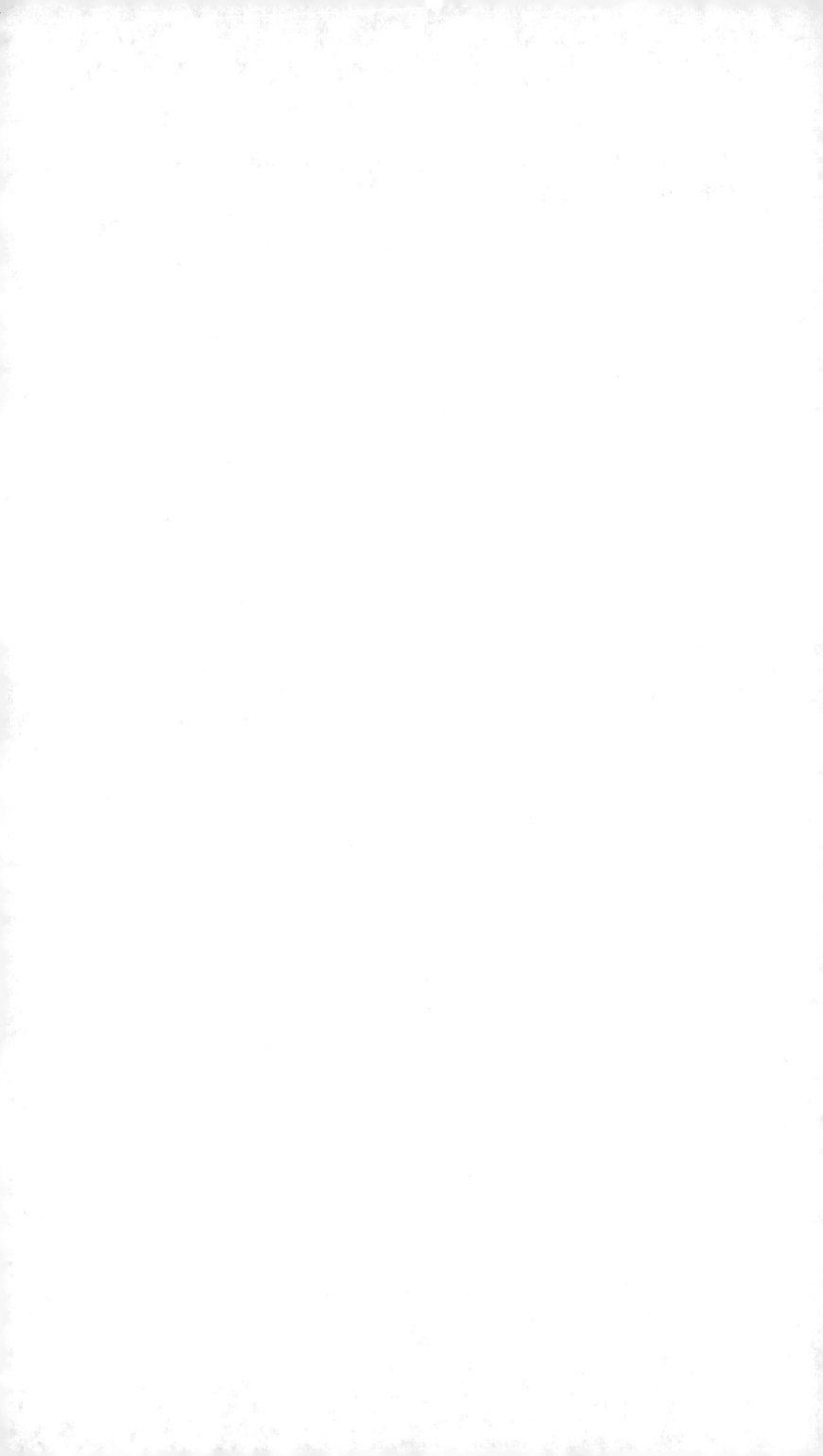

Conclusion

Thank you for reading this! We hope this short, concise book was able to teach you a thing or two about the intriguing HRT treatment.

Now that you understand the important factors regarding HRT, you can decide if you want to try it, or if you can inform your friends who ask you about it. Plus, a little addition to your knowledge doesn't hurt, right? Our world is becoming increasingly interested in the use of exogenous hormones, whether it be for sex changes, physical transformations, or as medical assistance to those who need it.

If you've learned anything from this book, please take the time to share your thoughts by sending me a personal message, or even posting a review on Amazon. It would be greatly appreciated and I try my best to get back to every message!

Thank you and good luck in your journey!